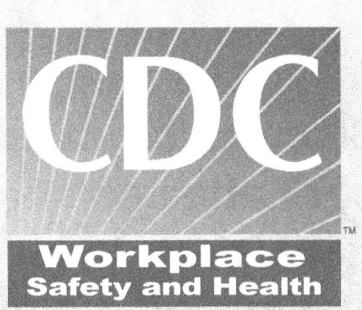

I0426173

Indoor Environmental Quality Evaluation at a Health Clinic – Indiana

Loren Tapp, MD, MS
Douglas Wiegand, PhD
Gregory Burr, CIH

Health Hazard Evaluation Report
HETA 2010-0168-3136
July 2011

DEPARTMENT OF HEALTH AND HUMAN SERVICES
Centers for Disease Control and Prevention

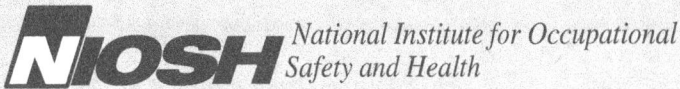 National Institute for Occupational Safety and Health

CONTENTS

ABBREVIATIONS

ASHRAE	American Society of Heating, Refrigerating and Air-Conditioning Engineers
HHE	Health hazard evaluation
HEPA	High-efficiency particulate air
HVAC	Heating, ventilating, and air-conditioning
IEQ	Indoor environmental quality
NAICS	North American Industry Classification System
NIOSH	National Institute for Occupational Safety and Health
ppm	Parts per million

The National Institute for Occupational Safety and Health (NIOSH) received a request from the Indiana Occupational Safety and Health Administration to evaluate a possible health hazard at a university-operated health clinic. Employees believed their symptoms were related to ongoing indoor environmental quality (IEQ) problems at the health clinic. Their symptoms included headache, dizziness, lethargy, cough, metallic tastes, and itchy and watery eyes.

What NIOSH Did

- We visited the health clinic on December 21, 2010.
- We looked for water damage, visible mold, and other IEQ problems.
- We measured carbon dioxide, temperature, and relative humidity in the clinic.
- We looked at the clinic's ventilation system.
- We looked at the findings from previous IEQ evaluations done at the clinic.
- We spoke to employees at the clinic privately.
- We reviewed the medical records of employees who had seen a doctor for work-related health concerns.

What NIOSH Found

- We did not see water damage to the walls, around exterior windows, or to the ceiling tiles.
- Temperature, relative humidity, and carbon dioxide levels in the clinic were within recommended guidelines.
- The ventilation system was in good condition and working well, despite its age.
- Odors from some second floor bathrooms could enter the health clinic.
- IEQ evaluations done at the clinic in 2008 and 2010 were thorough.
- Several employees reported having multiple symptoms when in the clinic. Many of these symptoms occurred when the building was being renovated.
- More than one third of employees believed that management was not adequately communicating to employees about possible workplace hazards.

What Managers Can Do

- Seal off areas of the building that are being renovated.
- Exhaust the second floor bathrooms to keep odors from entering the health clinic.

- Encourage employees to keep exterior windows closed to keep air that has not been filtered or controlled for humidity and temperature from entering the clinic.

- Encourage employees to report any health concerns that may be related to their work.

- Promptly address any concerns that employees report.

- Notify employees about what is being done to address their concerns and what future actions are being planned.

What Employees Can Do

- Keep exterior windows closed. Opening windows allows air that has not been filtered or controlled for humidity and temperature to enter the clinic.

- Report all health and safety concerns to managers.

- Seek care from an occupational health physician if you have physical symptoms related to your work.

- See a mental health specialist if you are having mental health symptoms related to your work.

SUMMARY

NIOSH was asked to evaluate employee concerns that were believed to be related to poor IEQ in a health clinic. We found the current IEQ satisfactory and noted improvements to the HVAC system; however, some clinic employees continued to report symptoms. We recommend sealing off building areas undergoing renovation, informing employees about these renovations, and promptly investigating work-related complaints reported by employees.

In response to a technical assistance request from the Indiana Occupational Safety and Health Administration we evaluated a university-operated health clinic on December 21, 2010. Employees of the health clinic believed that poor IEQ was responsible for symptoms including headache, dizziness, lethargy, itchy and watery eyes, cough, and a metallic taste. We measured carbon dioxide, temperature, and relative humidity in the health clinic throughout the workday. We looked for evidence of water damage and checked the HVAC system. We reviewed previous IEQ evaluations conducted by the university environmental health and safety office. We also held confidential interviews with employees to discuss their health and workplace concerns. Additionally, we reviewed the medical records from employees who saw a doctor because of work-related health concerns.

The carbon dioxide concentrations in the health clinic ranged from 475 to 600 ppm; outdoor concentrations were 420 ppm. Indoor carbon dioxide concentrations that are similar to outdoor concentrations suggest that the health clinic was adequately ventilated. Temperature in the health clinic ranged from 69°F–72°F, and relative humidity ranged from 22%–24%; these temperature and relative humidity levels are within recommended thermal comfort guidelines for the winter season. We did not see water damage to the walls, ceiling tiles, or exterior windows, and there was no evidence of water incursion in the space above the suspended ceiling. The constant volume HVAC system for the health clinic was approximately 40 years old but was well maintained. In 2010 the ventilation supply diffusers and return air grilles were cleaned, new thermostats were installed, and more outdoor air was provided to the HVAC system.

Sixteen of 22 employees who were interviewed reported having symptoms that began or worsened at work in the 2 months prior to our visit. The most commonly reported symptoms included headache, eye irritation, shortness of breath, chest tightness, fatigue, and dizziness. Most of the employees who reported experiencing symptoms in 2010 reported that they worsened during the second floor renovation, particularly during the cleaning and renovation of the pamphlet room. Most employees with work-related symptoms reported that their symptoms improved after renovation efforts on the second floor were completed. More than one third of the employees interviewed felt that management was not adequately communicating to employees what was being done to evaluate and resolve potential health hazards in the workplace.

A review of medical records from six employees found four employees with work-related symptoms that had begun or significantly worsened in April or May 2010. At that time, the building was undergoing renovations. Three of these four were diagnosed with an allergic illness exacerbated by working in the health clinic building. Records showed that the symptoms of these three employees had improved by their last medical visit.

We recommended that management maintain acceptable IEQ practices during renovation projects such as sealing off areas of the building that are being renovated. Management should also inform employees in advance about any remediation efforts, and track and promptly investigate any work-related complaints or problems reported by employees.

Keywords: NAICS 621498 (All other outpatient care centers), IEQ, carbon dioxide, temperature, relative humidity, ventilation, mold, health clinic, allergy symptoms

INTRODUCTION

NIOSH received a request for technical assistance in September 2010 from the Indiana Occupational Safety and Health Administration. The request concerned health clinic employees who reported that poor IEQ was responsible for symptoms including headache, dizziness, lethargy, itchy and watery eyes, coughing, and a metallic taste. An industrial hygienist from the university environmental health and safety office had completed two prior IEQ evaluations at this health clinic; however, employees were still reporting symptoms.

During our visit to the health clinic on December 21, 2010, we met with management and employees to discuss the request. We observed the health clinic layout and workplace conditions; measured carbon dioxide, temperature, and relative humidity; and held confidential interviews with employees. An interim letter dated February 9, 2011, was sent to management and employee representatives containing our preliminary findings and recommendations.

Background

The university-operated health clinic is located in a three story brick building constructed in 1937 and originally used as a hospital. The subbasement and third floor were unoccupied, and the basement and first floor contained administrative offices and clinical examination rooms. Most employees with health concerns worked on the second floor, which was the focus of this evaluation. The second floor contained offices, file rooms, and conference and meeting rooms. Approximately 30 employees, both part-time and full-time, worked on the second floor. The university planned to relocate the entire health clinic to a new building on the medical center campus by 2014 and then demolish this building.

Parts of the second floor of the health clinic building were renovated in 2010, including removing old wallpaper and carpet, preparing and painting walls, and installing new carpet. Clinic personnel reported that employee symptoms peaked during the summer of 2010, at which time renovations were actively proceeding.

ASSESSMENT

During a walk-through survey of the health clinic on December 21, 2010, we looked for evidence of water damage, water incursion, visible mold, and other potential IEQ problems. Measurements were taken in the morning and afternoon for carbon dioxide, temperature, and relative humidity using a Q-TRAK™ Plus Indoor Air Quality Monitor, Model 8554 (TSI Incorporated, Shoreview, Minnesota). We examined the constant volume HVAC system, including the type of air filters used and the location and condition of the outdoor air intakes. We used ventilation smoke tubes to evaluate air patterns in the health clinic and restrooms. We also reviewed reports of two IEQ evaluations (dated October 28, 2008, and June 24, 2010) that were prepared by the university environmental health and safety office.

We conducted confidential interviews with employees working on the first or second floors of the clinic who were present on the day of our site visit. The interview included questions on work history, medical history, and possible work-related symptoms. In addition, the interview covered employees' perceptions of health clinic management and communication, perceptions of whether a health hazard exists, and associated anxiety. We also requested medical records of employees who had seen a medical provider because of symptoms they felt were due to working in the health clinic building.

NIOSH Environmental Evaluation

We did not observe water damage to the walls, around exterior windows, or on the ceiling tiles, although reports of prior water damage and leaks had been mentioned by some clinic employees. We did not see evidence of water incursion or damage in the plenum (the space above the suspended ceiling). The second floor office space renovation was still underway. Two areas, Rooms 226 and 216, had been the main complaint areas before their renovation.

The carbon dioxide concentrations in the health clinic ranged from 495 to 585 ppm in the morning and from 475 to 600 ppm in the afternoon; outdoor concentrations were 420 ppm. We compared indoor and outdoor carbon dioxide concentrations to determine if indoor occupied spaces were adequately ventilated [ANSI/ASHRAE 2010a]. Because indoor and outdoor carbon dioxide concentrations were similar, the health clinic was determined to be adequately ventilated. Temperature in the health clinic ranged from 71°F–75°F, and relative humidity ranged from 21%–28%; these temperature and relative humidity values are within the ASHRAE recommended thermal comfort guidelines for the winter season [ANSI/ASHRAE 2010b]. The outdoor temperature ranged from 18°F–27°F with a relative humidity of approximately 20%.

The constant volume HVAC system serving the health clinic was about 40 years old and well maintained. The air handling unit used 1-inch thick pleated air filters (AAF Perfectpleat HCM8); these were correctly installed and changed quarterly. Individual 12-inch by 12-inch by 1-inch thick filters had been installed in many of the ceiling diffusers in the health clinic to capture any loose debris that may fall out of the ductwork; these filters were in good condition. In 2010 the university had installed new programmable Honeywell VisionPro® TH8000 thermostats, cleaned the supply diffusers and return air grilles, and provided additional outdoor air to the HVAC system at the health clinic. An industrial hygienist for the university environmental health and safety office estimated that 25% more outdoor air was now provided to the HVAC system.

Although exterior windows in the health clinic could be opened by employees, none were open during this evaluation. It is preferable not to open windows in a commercial office because this permits unconditioned and unfiltered air to enter the area and may make it more difficult to maintain good IEQ. In June 2010, the health clinic management offered employees (upon request) Honeywell Model F113A6001 commercial grade portable air cleaners. These air cleaners, equipped with both HEPA and sorbent (charcoal) filters, were intended to help address employee's concerns about the air quality. We looked at two of these portable air cleaners, and both appeared in excellent condition and well maintained.

In response to employee concerns about the drinking water quality, the health clinic management arranged to test the water for lead; results were within acceptable guidelines. In addition to the water testing, water fountains in the health clinic were filtered with equipment provided and maintained by Pure Water Tech LLC, Indianapolis, Indiana.

Using ventilation smoke tubes, we found that three of the four second floor restrooms (Rooms 206, 207, and 233) were under positive pressure in relation to the health clinic (meaning that air would flow out from the restroom and into the surrounding area). This situation may allow nuisance odors from the restrooms to migrate into the health clinic. The custodial closet where housekeeping chemicals and equipment were stored was properly kept under negative pressure (air flowed into the custodial closet from the surrounding area).

NIOSH Medical Evaluation

Employee Interviews

We held confidential interviews with 22 of 24 employees who were present on the day of our site visit. Of the 22 interviewed employees, 16 were female, the average age was 43 years (range from 28 to 66 years), and the average number of years worked at the health clinic was 7 years (range from 9 months to 14 years). Seventeen of the 22 employees worked mainly on the second floor, and the remaining five employees worked mainly on the first floor. Two of 22 employees reported being current smokers at the time of the evaluation; seven reported smoking in the past. Nine reported taking allergy or asthma medication, four reported a history of asthma, and three reported a history of allergic rhinitis.

Reported Symptoms

Sixteen of the 22 employees interviewed reported having health problems that began or worsened at work, 12 from the second floor and 4 from the first floor. When asked about specific symptoms at work within the 2 months prior to our visit, employees reported experiencing headache (14), eye irritation (12), dizziness (10), shortness of breath (10), chest tightness (10), fatigue (10), nose irritation (9), cough (9), throat irritation (7), body aches (7), and wheeze (5). Symptoms that were reported by five or fewer employees included metallic taste, nausea, earache or ear infection, vertigo or feeling "off balance," pneumonia, rash, and angioedema (tissue swelling just below the skin). Ten employees reported that their symptoms improved when they left the building and worsened when they re-entered the building. When asked what they thought caused their symptoms, eight employees reported mold. Other causes, each reported by three or fewer employees, were "something in the building," renovation/demolition particles, dust and dirt in the building, "stuff from the vents," "something in the pamphlet room," seasonal pollen, roach allergens, and asbestos. Three of the 16 employees reporting symptoms were moved to a different work location (out of the building or to a different floor); two of the 16 took a medical leave of absence; and 8 of the 16 reported seeing a medical provider for their symptoms.

Health clinic employees reported that allergy and mild respiratory symptoms had been going on for years because of alleged mold and dust in the building. Several employees reported having a history of allergy or sinus problems. Most of the employees who reported symptoms in 2010 said the symptoms worsened during the second floor renovation, particularly during the cleaning and renovation of the pamphlet room. Almost all interviewed employees reported experiencing some upper respiratory irritation for 1 or 2 days during the peak of the renovation activities involving the central section of the second floor. First floor employees reported that their symptoms worsened when they entered the second floor. Some employees also reported that the second floor walls were "black with mold" when the old wallpaper was removed.

Psychosocial Evaluation

Most employees believed management was dedicated to resolving issues related to health hazards in the workplace. Examples given were providing portable air cleaners and cleaning the ventilation ductwork. Other employees were more critical, believing that management should have acted more quickly in response to initial employee concerns and that more could be done to address and remedy the perceived poor IEQ.

Three quarters of the employees interviewed agreed that management was approachable regarding work-related health concerns. Other employees disagreed, believing that it was best to not speak up for fear of being patronized or reassigned and that nothing would be done to address their concern. One third of the employees described a lack of two-way communication between management and employees regarding health and safety issues in the workplace.

All employees interviewed reported that they were aware that coworkers were experiencing health issues believed to be workplace related. A majority reported that they heard of their coworkers' health issues through informal discussions with other employees. Five individuals reported learning of the issues from management.

Over one third of the employees interviewed believed that management was not adequately communicating to employees what was being done to evaluate and resolve potential health hazards in the workplace. To evaluate this in more detail, we asked several questions regarding the two IEQ evaluations performed on the second floor of the building in 2008 and 2010.

Fifteen of the interviewed employees were not aware of the evaluation by the university environmental health and safety office in October 2008. Of the seven who were aware of this evaluation, all were working at the clinic at the time of the evaluation. However, five of the seven did not know the outcome. All but one employee were made aware of the second evaluation by the environmental health and safety office in June 2010 following an office meeting or from their supervisor. Although several employees were unaware of the outcome of the evaluation, nearly half reported that nothing of concern was found. Nearly a quarter reported that the outcome involved management following recommendations to clean areas and provide air filters to improve IEQ.

Seventeen of the 22 interviewed employees believed they were exposed to a health hazard while at work. However, when these

17 individuals were asked to rate their anxiety level associated with their exposure beliefs on a scale from 1 ("no anxiety") to 10 ("a great deal of anxiety") the average response was 3.5, with half of the individuals reporting "no anxiety."

Medical Record Review

Six of seven employees' medical records were received and reviewed. Three employees were seen by the university occupational health clinic and three by their primary care provider. Two employees were referred to an allergist, one by occupational health and one by the primary care provider. These two employees underwent allergy testing; one was found to be allergic to dust mites, multiple molds, and cockroach antigens; the other employee was not allergic to any of the tested materials. Records from two other employees documented allergies by prior allergy testing. Of the six employees' medical records we reviewed, two did not contain information about work-related symptoms. The four remaining records contained doctors' notes indicating that their symptoms were related to working in the building, and three documented symptoms but no specific diagnoses for headache, dizziness, and/or nausea in addition to allergic symptoms. The physicians noted that the employees' symptoms had begun or significantly worsened in April or May 2010 during building renovations. Diagnoses included allergic rhinitis, asthma, urticaria (hives), and nonallergic chronic rhinitis. Three of the four employees with work-related symptoms had improved by the time of their last medical visit.

Previous Health Clinic Evaluations

In the IEQ report dated October 28, 2008, an industrial hygienist from the university environmental health and safety office evaluated symptoms of watery eyes, burning nose, chest tightness, and a "dirt taste" in the mouth among employees in the health clinic. Employees associated their symptoms with an unknown odor from the HVAC system when the heat was first switched on for the fall season. The industrial hygienist measured carbon dioxide, temperature, and relative humidity levels within recommended guidelines and levels of particulates and volatile organic compounds in the health clinic that were lower than outdoor levels. Recommendations included opening the HVAC outdoor air intake, cleaning the return air grilles, purchasing portable air cleaners equipped with both HEPA and sorbent (charcoal) filters, and switching the HVAC system from cooling to heating mode when the health clinic was unoccupied to minimize employees smelling any transient nuisance odors.

In the June 24, 2010, IEQ report, the levels of carbon dioxide, temperature, and relative humidity remained within recommended guidelines, and levels of particulates and volatile organic compounds in the health clinic were lower than outdoor levels. The industrial hygienist identified several nonfunctioning thermostats, observed dirty return air grilles, detected a slight odor in Room 222 (and noted that the supply diffuser for this room was closed), and found the wood paneling beneath an exterior window bulging from possible water damage. Recommendations included cleaning the return air grilles, investigating and repairing the window leak, and repairing or replacing the nonfunctioning thermostats.

DISCUSSION

Despite satisfactory IEQ measurements and improvements to the health clinic's HVAC system, some employees continued to report symptoms. We have learned from conducting numerous IEQ evaluations that the multitude of symptoms reported by building occupants can be wide ranging and are neither suggestive of any particular medical diagnosis nor readily associated with a causative agent. Reports demonstrate closer associations of symptom occurrence with occupant perceptions of the indoor environment rather than with any measurement of indoor contaminants or conditions [Berglund and Cain 1989; NIOSH 1991]. A typical spectrum of reported symptoms includes headaches, fatigue, itching or burning eyes, skin irritation, nasal congestion, dry or irritated throats, and other respiratory symptoms. These symptoms are also often experienced by people outside of the workplace and could be related to a number of different causes, such as respiratory infections, allergies, discomfort due to temperature and humidity, and stress. Some studies have shown that psychological, social, and organizational factors may modify individuals' and organizations' responses to concerns in the office environment [Baker 1989; Boxer 1990; Ooi and Goh 1997]. Typically, employees suspect a workplace cause because their symptoms appear to be worse while at work and better when away from work. In this evaluation, medical records review found three employees diagnosed with an allergic illness exacerbated by working in the health clinic building.

Generally, we look for water damage to determine if a building has a mold problem. In the June 2010 IEQ report by the university environmental health and safety office, some potential water damage to the building was identified. It is possible that in the spring and summer of 2010, as old carpeting and wallpaper were removed, mold spores were released into the air.

Allergic responses are the most common type of health problem associated with exposure to molds. Symptoms may include sneezing; itching of the nose, eyes, mouth, or throat; nasal stuffiness and runny nose; and red, itchy eyes. Repeated or single exposure to mold or mold spores may cause previously nonsensitized individuals to become sensitized. Molds can trigger asthma symptoms (shortness of breath, wheezing, cough) in persons who are allergic to mold. The types and severity of symptoms related to exposure to mold in the indoor environment depend in part on the extent of the mold present, the extent of the individual's exposure, and the susceptibility of the individual (for example, whether he or she has preexisting allergies or asthma). For more information see Appendix A.

DISCUSSION

(CONTINUED)

Information gathered during interviews suggests that some employees were not comfortable approaching management with a health or safety related concern, and one third of employees believed that two-way communication between employees and management on health and safety issues was lacking. It may be helpful to develop methods in which employees can voice their concerns to management and feel involved by offering solutions. Examples include forming a health and safety committee where employees can express their concerns in a forum setting, designating a volunteer liaison between employees and management, and implementing an anonymous feedback program where employees can bring attention to issues or offer suggestions.

One third of the employees believed that they were not receiving adequate information from management regarding how potential hazards in the health clinic were being addressed. Employees reported that much of the information they received regarding potential exposures and management's efforts to address them were based on office gossip. Such informal communication can result in mixed messages, rumors, or other misinformation which can negatively affect workplace stress, frustration, and trust in management [Boxer 1990].

Nearly 80% of the employees interviewed believe they were exposed to a health hazard at work, yet most reported a low level of anxiety associated with it. This may indicate that many of the employees did not believe it was a serious issue, or the symptoms they experienced (if any) were not severe. Nonetheless, several employees reported experiencing a high level of anxiety due to their belief that they were being exposed to a health hazard at work.

The psychosocial aspect of our evaluation focused on communication issues and perceptions of risk. Other psychosocial variables related to job stress (e.g., job satisfaction, interpersonal conflict, and lack of job security) are often associated with workplaces where IEQ issues are of concern [Kreiss 1989; Boxer 1990; Norbäck et al. 1990; Godish 1995; Ooi and Goh 1997]. Job stress is associated with a variety of negative health-related outcomes [WHO 2010], and thus it may be helpful to assess these issues in more detail.

CONCLUSIONS

Overall, we found that the current status of the IEQ of the health clinic was good during this evaluation. We saw no evidence of current water leaks or water damage, and the HVAC system was functioning properly. However, many employees reported allergic and other symptoms that worsened while working inside the clinic building. Most of the employees who reported experiencing symptoms in 2010 said their symptoms began or worsened during the second floor renovation, particularly the cleaning and renovation of the pamphlet room. Medical records review found three employees diagnosed with an allergic illness exacerbated by working in the health clinic building. Although most employees' symptoms have improved since the renovations have slowed, a few employees continued to have symptoms. About one third of employees interviewed were not satisfied with management's efforts to solve the problem or with management's communication with employees regarding the issue.

RECOMMENDATIONS

Since 1972, NIOSH has conducted more than 1,250 HHEs related to IEQ. We have found that significant IEQ improvements can be achieved by following standard recommendations related to four areas:

1. Operation and maintenance of ventilation system and other building components
2. Remediation of moisture, mold, and odor problems
3. Addressing employee issues through administrative controls
4. Expanding opportunities for employees to participate in decision making

On the basis of our findings, we recommend the actions listed below to create a more healthful workplace. We encourage the management of the health clinic to use a labor-management health and safety committee or working group to discuss the recommendations in this report and develop an action plan. Those involved in the work can best set priorities and assess the feasibility of our recommendations for the specific situation at the health clinic. Our recommendations are based on the hierarchy of controls approach. This approach groups actions by their likely effectiveness in reducing or removing hazards. In most cases, the preferred approach is to eliminate hazardous materials or processes and install engineering controls to reduce exposure or shield employees. Until such controls are in place, or if they are not effective or feasible, administrative measures may be needed.

Engineering Controls

Engineering controls reduce exposures to employees by removing the hazard from the process or placing a barrier between the hazard and the employee. Engineering controls are very effective at protecting employees without placing primary responsibility of implementation on the employee.

1. Adjust the exhaust ventilation in the second floor bathrooms to make sure they are maintained under negative pressure when the clinic is occupied [ANSI/ASHRAE 2010a].

Administrative Controls

Administrative controls are management-dictated work practices and policies to reduce or prevent exposures to workplace hazards. The effectiveness of administrative changes in work practices for controlling workplace hazards is dependent on management commitment and employee acceptance. Regular monitoring and reinforcement are necessary to ensure that control policies and procedures are not circumvented in the name of convenience or production.

1. Follow good practice guidelines for maintaining acceptable IEQ during construction and renovation projects. This includes scheduling renovation activities and informing employees in advance about any remediation efforts such as removal of carpeting or wallpaper. For detailed information, see Appendix B: "Good Practice Guidelines for Maintaining Acceptable Indoor Environmental Quality During Construction and Renovation Projects."

2. Discourage employees from opening exterior windows because this allows unconditioned and unfiltered air to enter, making maintaining good IEQ more difficult.

3. Improve communication between management and employees regarding responses to employee health and

safety concerns. A supervisor or manager who is sensitive to the employees' concerns should communicate directly with those who report health and safety concerns. Points to consider include:

a. Actively listening to employees' concerns in a nonjudgmental manner. Employees should feel that their concerns are taken seriously.

b. Regularly informing employees of exactly what steps are being taken to assess the problem, what has been determined, and what remains to be determined. A combination of written reports and face-to-face meetings is valuable.

c. Routinely share information with employees rather than waiting until a definitive cause of the problem is discovered; this will reduce the chance of distorted information.

4. Track and investigate work-related complaints or problems reported by employees, and share the findings with employees.

5. Encourage employees with health concerns related to their workplace to seek evaluation and care from a physician who is residency trained and/or board certified in occupational medicine and is familiar with the types of exposures employees may have had and their health effects. The Association of Occupational and Environmental Clinics (http://www.aoec.org) and the American College of Occupational and Environmental Medicine (http://www.acoem.org) maintain lists of their members.

6. Encourage employees experiencing symptoms of anxiety (e.g., persistent troubling thoughts, fatigue, difficulty concentrating, or irritability) related to their working environment to seek mental health services to address such symptoms if they are interfering with social, occupational, or other important areas of functioning.

7. Consider having an expert assess the psychosocial and job stress issues and make recommendations for remedial actions, if needed.

REFERENCES

ANSI/ASHRAE [2010a]. Ventilation for acceptable indoor air quality. American National Standards Institute/ASHRAE standard 62.1–2010. Atlanta, GA: American Society of Heating, Refrigerating, and Air-Conditioning Engineers, Inc.

ANSI/ASHRAE [2010b]. Thermal environmental conditions for human occupancy. American National Standards Institute/ASHRAE standard 55-2010. Atlanta, GA: American Society for Heating, Refrigerating, and Air-Conditioning Engineers, Inc.

Baker DB [1989]. Social and organizational factors in office building associated illness. Occup Med: State of the Art Reviews 4(4):607–624.

Berglund L, Cain WS [1989]. Perceived air quality and the thermal environment. In: Proceedings of IAQ '89: The Human Equation: Health and Comfort. Atlanta, GA: American Society of Heating, Ventilating, and Air-Conditioning Engineers, pp. 93–99.

Boxer PA [1990]. Indoor air quality: a psychosocial perspective. J Occup Med 32(5):425–428.

Godish T [1995]. Sick buildings: Definition, diagnosis, and mitigation. Boca Raton, FL: CRC Press.

Kreiss K [1989]. The epidemiology of building-related complaints and illness. Occup Med: State of the Art Reviews 4(4):575–592.

NIOSH [1991]. Hazard evaluation and technical assistance report: Library of Congress, Washington. D.C. Cincinnati, OH: U.S. Department of Health and Human Services, Public Health Service, Centers for Disease Control, National Institute for Occupational Safety and Health, NIOSH Report No. HHE 88–364-2104.

Norbäck D, Michel I, Widstrom J [1990]. Indoor air quality and personal factors related to the sick building syndrome. Scan J Work Environ Health 16(2):121–128.

Ooi PL, Goh KT [1997]. Sick building syndrome: an emerging stress-related disorder? Int J Epidemiol 26(6):1243–1249.

WHO [2010]. Health impact of psychosocial hazards at work. Geneva: Switzerland. [http://whqlibdoc.who.int/publications/2010/9789241500272_eng.pdf]. Date accessed: June 2011.

Exposure to microbes is not unique to the indoor environment. No environment, indoors or out, is completely free from microbes. Remediation of microbial contamination may improve IEQ conditions even though a specific cause-effect relationship is not determined. NIOSH investigators routinely recommend the remediation of observed microbial contamination and the correction of situations that are favorable for microbial growth and bioaerosol dissemination.

The types and severity of symptoms related to exposure to mold in the indoor environment depend in part on the extent of the mold present, the extent of the individual's exposure, and the susceptibility of the individual (for example, whether he or she has pre-existing allergies or asthma). In general, excessive exposure to fungi may produce health problems by several primary mechanisms, including allergy or hypersensitivity, infection, and toxic effects. Additionally, molds produce a variety of volatile organic compounds, the most common of which is ethanol, that have been postulated to cause upper airway irritation. Evidence also shows that exposure to fungal fragments that can contain allergens, toxins, and $(1\rightarrow3)$-β-D-glucan may occur [Górny et al. 2002; Brasel et al. 2005; Reponen et al. 2006].

Allergic responses are the most common type of health problem associated with mold exposure. These health problems may include sneezing; itching of the nose, eyes, mouth, or throat; nasal stuffiness and runny nose; and red, itchy eyes. Repeated or single exposure to mold or mold spores may cause previously nonsensitized individuals to become sensitized. Molds can trigger asthma symptoms (shortness of breath, wheezing, cough) in persons who are allergic to mold. In the 2004 report, "Damp Indoor Spaces and Health," the Institute of Medicine found sufficient evidence of an association between mold or dampness indoors and nasal and throat symptoms, asthma symptoms in sensitized asthmatics, wheeze, cough, and hypersensitivity pneumonitis in susceptible persons [IOM 2004], and limited or suggestive evidence of an association between lower respiratory illness in healthy children and damp indoor spaces. Evidence was inadequate or insufficient to determine whether an association exists between dyspnea (shortness of breath), airflow obstruction in healthy persons, mucous membrane irritation, skin symptoms, chronic obstructive pulmonary disease, asthma development, inhalation fevers in nonoccupational settings, fatigue, cancer, reproductive effects, neuropsychiatric effects, lower respiratory illness in healthy adults, gastrointestinal problems, rheumatologic or immune problems, or acute idiopathic pulmonary hemorrhage in infants. No health conditions met the level of evidence for causation.

In 2009, the World Health Organization published guidelines for protection of public health from mold and other exposures in damp buildings [WHO 2009]. On the basis of its review of the scientific literature for this report, they concluded that there was sufficient epidemiologic evidence that occupants of damp buildings are at risk of developing upper and lower respiratory tract symptoms (including cough, wheeze, and shortness of breath), respiratory infections, asthma, and exacerbation of asthma. The World Health Organization also concluded that limited evidence suggested an association between bronchitis and allergic rhinitis and damp buildings and noted clinical evidence that exposure to mold and other microbial agents in damp buildings is associated with hypersensitivity pneumonitis.

People with weakened immune systems (immune-compromised or immune-suppressed individuals) may be more vulnerable to infections by molds. For example, *Aspergillus fumigatus* is a fungal species that has been found almost everywhere on every conceivable type of substrate. It has been known to infect the lungs of immune-compromised individuals after inhalation of the airborne spores [Wald and Stave 1994; Brandt et al. 2006]. Healthy individuals are usually not vulnerable to infections from airborne mold exposure.

No exposure guidelines for mold in air exist, so it is not possible to distinguish between "safe" and "unsafe" levels of exposure. Nevertheless, the potential for health problems is an important reason to prevent indoor mold growth and to remediate any indoor mold contamination. Moisture intrusion, along with nutrient sources such as building materials or furnishings, allows mold to grow indoors, so it is important to keep the building interior and furnishings dry. NIOSH agrees with the U.S. Environmental Protection Agency's recommendations to remedy mold contamination in indoor environments (http://www.epa.gov/mold/mold_remediation.html) [U.S. EPA 2001; Redd SC 2002]. Additional information on health effects and mold remediation can be found in the Center for Disease Control and Prevention document "Mold Prevention Strategies and Possible Health Effects in the Aftermath of Hurricanes and Major Floods" at http://www.cdc.gov/mmwr/preview/mmwrhtml/rr5508a1.htm.

References

Brandt M, Brown C, Burkhart J, Burton N, Cox-Ganser J, Damon S, Falk H, Fridkin S, Garbe P, McGeehin M, Morgan J, Page E, Rao C, Redd S, Sinks T, Trout D, Wallingford K, Warnock D, Weissman D [2006]. Mold prevention strategies and possible health effects in the aftermath of hurricanes and major floods. MMWR 55(RR-8):1–27.

Brasel T, Martin J, Carriker C, Wilson S, Straus D [2005]. Detection of airborne Stachybotrys chartarum macrocyclic trichothecene mycotoxins in the indoor environment. Appl Environ Microbiol 71(11):7376–7388.

Górny R, Reponen T, Willeke K, Schmechel D, Robine E, Boissier M, Grinshpun SA [2002]. Fungal fragments as indoor air biocontaminants. Appl Environ Microbiol 68(7):3522–3531.

IOM [2004]. Human health effects associated with damp indoor environments. In: Damp indoor spaces and health. Washington, DC: Institute of Medicine, National Academy Press, pp. 183–269.

Redd S [2002]. State of the science on molds and human health. Statement for the Record Before the Subcommittee on Oversight and Investigations and Housing and Community Opportunity, Committee on Financial Services, United States House of Representatives. Atlanta, GA: U.S. Department of Health and Human Services, Centers for Disease Control and Prevention.

Reponen T, Seo S-C, Iossifova Y, Adhikari A, Grinshpun SA [2006]. New field-compatible method for collection and analysis of β-glucan in fungal fragments. Abstracts of the International Aerosol Conference, St. Paul, Minnesota, p. 955.

U.S. EPA [2001]. Mold remediation in schools and commercial buildings. Washington, DC: United States Environmental Protection Agency, Office of Air and Radiation, Indoor Environments Division. EPA Publication No. 402-K-01-001.

Wald P, Stave G [1994]. Fungi. In: Physical and biological hazards of the workplace. New York: Van Nostrand Reinhold, p. 394.

WHO [2009]. WHO guidelines for indoor air quality: dampness and mould. Geneva, Switzerland: World Health Organization. [http://www.euro.who.int/document/e92645.pdf]. Date accessed: June 2011.

Introduction

The following good practice guidelines for maintaining acceptable IEQ during construction and renovation projects were prepared to serve as objective criteria for the evaluation of building construction and renovation practices by NIOSH. They are also intended to be educational and informative. These guidelines were prepared from information contained in two reference documents along with our own collective experience. These two reference documents are "IAQ Guidelines for Occupied Buildings Under Construction," prepared and published by the Sheet Metal and Air-Conditioning Contractors' National Association, Inc. [SMACNA 1995] and "Construction/ Renovation Influence on Indoor Air Quality" an article published in the October 1996 issue of the ASHRAE Journal [Kuehn 1996].

Background

Construction and renovation projects can adversely affect building occupants by the release of airborne dusts, gases, organic vapors, and odors during construction, renovation, demolition, repair, or reconfiguration activities. Microbiological contaminants can also be released during construction and renovation activities. Two sources of contaminants, those generated from inside the building and those generated from outside the building, need to be considered. There are several important distinctions regarding exposures of construction workers versus exposures of nonconstruction workers (building occupants), and these differences are critically important in the development of management strategies to (1) ensure awareness on the part of the construction contractors regarding the potential impact of construction and renovation activities on building occupants, (2) anticipate construction and renovation activities that may generate contaminants, and (3) implement controls to minimize or prevent exposures of both construction and renovation workers and building occupants. Foresight and planning are necessary prerequisites to prevent IEQ-related complaints during building construction and renovation activities. Even nuisance odors and dusts from construction and renovation activities can be triggering factors, resulting in complaints from building occupants. These complaints can be due to actual symptoms resulting from exposures or to a perceived risk of exposures to unknown materials, which may or may not be an actual health hazard.

Effective maintenance of acceptable IEQ during construction and renovation activities requires a collective effort and input from building managers, the general contractor, subcontractors, engineers, and building occupants. Input from HVAC professionals and architects is important to assess ventilation system performance when making design changes or implementing control measures. The ability and desire for effective communication between all parties is essential, especially during rapidly changing circumstances, which are often a hallmark of construction- and renovation-related activities.

Guidelines for Initial Planning

During the initial stages of any construction or renovation activity is the appropriate time to develop a site- and activity-specific plan to control contaminants that may affect construction or renovation workers and building occupants.

- Identify all key personnel (representatives from the building and general contractor) responsible for addressing construction- or renovation-related activities and airborne contaminant control. Other personnel such as building staff, engineers, and subcontractors, should be involved as necessary.

- Develop a construction or renovation impact assessment describing anticipated work activities, along with their associated source contaminants, generation points, and areas potentially affected by the release of air contaminants.

- Develop a detailed budget for the contaminant control methods to be utilized.

Guidelines for Bid Specifications

Bid document specifications should be developed. In addition to general control measures, the bid document should include the particular control measures appropriate for the specific construction or renovation project being proposed. These bid specifications should be clearly written to reduce the likelihood of misinterpretation.

- Identify the specific controls needed for the construction or renovation project along with the appropriate performance metrics, and write specifications into the bid document accordingly.

- Require the general contractor to designate a representative to handle IEQ issues and establish appropriate channels of communication with subcontractors.

- Specify construction or renovation conditions that would require an emergency response (such as a contaminant release into an occupied area).

Guidelines for Control Options

Because a variety of methods are available for the control of indoor- and outdoor-generated contaminants, the most effective and cost efficient strategies should be considered for implementation.

- Schedule construction or renovation work during periods of low building occupancy or low occupancy adjacent to the work areas, if possible.

- Isolate work areas from occupied areas using critical barriers, negative and positive pressurization, and HEPA filtration, as necessary, and minimize the number of building penetrations required for the construction or renovation activities.

- Negatively pressurize work areas and/or positively pressurize occupied areas to prevent migration of air contaminants from work areas to occupied areas.

- Modify HVAC operations as necessary during times of construction or renovation activities to ensure isolation of work areas from occupied areas. This could include increasing the HVAC outdoor air intake filtration efficiency and temporarily relocating the HVAC outdoor air intakes serving the occupied areas.

- Maintain an adequate unoccupied buffer zone around the work areas to allow for construction or renovation traffic and to ensure acceptable IEQ. This could require temporarily relocating building occupants closest to the work areas.

- Increase housekeeping activities in adjacent occupied areas during construction or renovation projects.

- Specify low-emitting materials for use in construction or renovation projects to reduce the likelihood of contaminant generation.

Guidelines to Protect HVAC Systems

Protect the HVAC system(s) serving the construction or renovation areas from damage or contamination.

- Disable the HVAC system(s) serving the construction or renovation areas, if possible.

- Isolate portions of the HVAC system where appropriate to prevent damage or contamination.

- Block or seal return air grilles in construction or renovation areas.

- Upgrade filtration efficiency in the HVAC systems continuing in use during construction or renovation activities.

- Do not store construction materials or equipment in HVAC mechanical rooms.

Guidelines for Good Work Practices

Good work and housekeeping practices that minimize contaminant release and ensure acceptable IEQ are essential to the success of any construction or renovation project.

- Use local exhaust ventilation with HEPA filtration where dust generation is anticipated. If local exhaust is not feasible, portable air cleaning devices could be used as appropriate.

- Use work practices and materials that result in little or no generation of airborne contaminants during construction or renovation activities, such as wet methods to suppress dust generation.

- Identify routes for construction or renovation traffic through unoccupied areas and away from building openings to occupied areas.

- Use HEPA vacuums and damp mop regularly to clean floors and ledges during construction or renovation activities.

- Bag and promptly remove off site all construction or renovation debris through demolition chutes on the exterior of building and/or through other dedicated perimeter wall penetrations.

- Locate dumpsters and salvage bins away from operating HVAC outdoor air intakes and exterior doors to occupied areas.

Guidelines to Implement Project Specifications (Heading 1)

Effective implementation and management of the construction or renovation project are essential to maintain acceptable IEQ for the building occupants.

- Ensure that the general contractor's IEQ designee is adequately trained and has the authority to immediately correct problems affecting IEQ as they arise.

- Hold regular meetings between building representatives, the general contractor, subcontractors, and other personnel as appropriate to ensure acceptable IEQ.

- Monitor construction or renovation activities carefully so that all work conforms to the bid document specifications.

- Monitor the pressurization of construction or renovation and occupied areas to ensure that the complete isolation of the work area is maintained.

- Monitor for airborne contaminants in the occupied areas as appropriate to ensure acceptable IEQ.

Guidelines to Maintain Effective Communication

Ensure that effective communication exists between building occupants, the project manager, the general contractor, subcontractors, and other personnel as appropriate.

- Prior to the start of construction or renovation activities, communicate the scope of work and the precautions that will be used to control the release of contaminants.

- Update building occupants regarding the project's progress and other pertinent information during the construction or renovation project.

- Respond promptly to IEQ complaints from building occupants regarding construction or renovation issues and specify any situations requiring an emergency response.

Guidelines to Commission Work Area

- Use 100% outdoor air to ventilate the work areas before and during initial occupancy.

- Test and balance the HVAC system(s) in the work areas, preferably before occupancy.

- Monitor for airborne contaminants in the work areas (as necessary) to ensure acceptable IEQ during initial occupancy.

References

SMACNA [1995]. IAQ guidelines for occupied buildings under construction. Chantilly, VA: Sheet Metal and Air Conditioning Contractors' National Association, Inc.

Kuehn T [1996]. Construction/renovation influence on indoor air quality. ASHRAE Journal 38(10):22–29.

Acknowledgments and Availability of Report

The Hazard Evaluations and Technical Assistance Branch (HETAB) of the National Institute for Occupational Safety and Health (NIOSH) conducts field investigations of possible health hazards in the workplace. These investigations are conducted under the authority of Section 20(a)(6) of the Occupational Safety and Health Act of 1970, 29 U.S.C. 669(a)(6) which authorizes the Secretary of Health and Human Services, following a written request from any employer or authorized representative of employees, to determine whether any substance normally found in the place of employment has potentially toxic effects in such concentrations as used or found. HETAB also provides, upon request, technical and consultative assistance to federal, state, and local agencies; labor; industry; and other groups or individuals to control occupational health hazards and to prevent related trauma and disease.

Mention of any company or product does not constitute endorsement by NIOSH. In addition, citations to websites external to NIOSH do not constitute NIOSH endorsement of the sponsoring organizations or their programs or products. Furthermore, NIOSH is not responsible for the content of these websites. All Web addresses referenced in this document were accessible as of the publication date.

This report was prepared by Loren Tapp, Douglas Wiegand, and Gregory Burr of HETAB, Division of Surveillance, Hazard Evaluations and Field Studies. Health communication assistance was provided by Stefanie Evans. Editorial assistance was provided by Ellen Galloway. Desktop publishing was performed by Robin Smith.

Copies of this report have been sent to employee and management representatives at the health clinic, the Indiana Occupational Safety and Health Administration office requesting the technical assistance, the university environmental health and safety department, the state health department, and the Occupational Safety and Health Administration Regional Office. This report is not copyrighted and may be freely reproduced. The report may be viewed and printed at http://www.cdc.gov/niosh/hhe/. Copies may be purchased from the National Technical Information Service at 5825 Port Royal Road, Springfield, Virginia 22161.

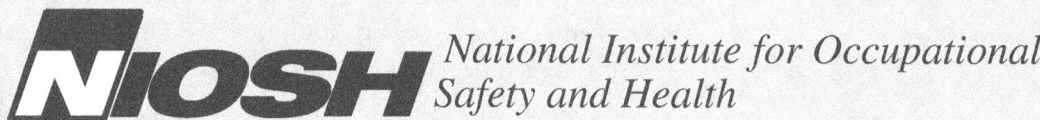

National Institute for Occupational Safety and Health

Delivering on the Nation's promise: Safety and health at work for all people through research and prevention.

To receive NIOSH documents or information about occupational safety and health topics, contact NIOSH at:

1-800-CDC-INFO (1-800-232-4636)

TTY: 1-888-232-6348

E-mail: cdcinfo@cdc.gov

or visit the NIOSH web site at: **www.cdc.gov/niosh.**

For a monthly update on news at NIOSH, subscribe to NIOSH eNews by visiting **www.cdc.gov/niosh/eNews.**

SAFER • HEALTHIER • PEOPLE™